THE ADVENTURES OF REESE AND RUFUS

The Adventures of Reese and Rufus

The Day Reese and Rufus Met

BY ALITA-GERI CARTER, MSN, RN, CPNP-PC

Illustrator: Jarrad Crutcher

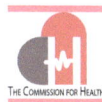

The Commission for Health

First Printing, 2020
Library of Congress Control Number: 2020918977

To every child that reads this book,
Your life is important and you were
created to do great things. You are loved.
May your joy, strength, and determination
continue to inspire us all.

Author: Alita-Geri Carter, MSN, RN, CPNP-PC
Illustrator: Jarrad Crutcher

Acknowledgments

To the Ones who Made this Possible,

I would like to give a special thank you to my editors Candice P. Stewart, and Deanna M. Vaughn. Thank you to my legal advisor, mentor, and sister Sharnae Smith for pushing me to write these stories. Thank you, Mr. Crutcher, for you bringing our story to life and for your dedication. I would like to say thank you to my husband who faced many frightening and heart-breaking experiences with me. Only the parental figures and caregivers of a child with needs will understand the heartache or heartbreak of what it means to have a child with special and/or medical needs. Our hearts have ached repeatedly over the years, **but God** has been good to us.

To our Supporters,

Thank you! Our books are based upon our family's real-life experiences. We have overcome many obstacles as a family. We hope that by sharing her stories in these books that other children and families know that they are not alone and that there is hope for a better day. When Reese was younger, she was ill often. As a family, we had to learn how to be brave together and how to face hard moments together (like spending the holiday in urgent care, staying overnight in an emergency room, or being admitted to a hospital). At the time of this book being published, our daughter has had many visits to the emergency room, received care from a number of specialists, had a hospital admission, two surgeries, one failed surgery attempt, multiple evaluations, and varying types of therapies. During these times, Reese has shown us what it means to be brave, and unstoppable. She never ceases to amaze us.

To our Village,

I would like to thank you for the support you have provided to our family over the years. To my mother, closest friends, and counselors, thank you for taking this journey with us and carrying us when we did not have the strength to walk this journey alone. Most of all we thank you Jesus for keeping our family safe and covering us with your grace.

Reese,

I would like to thank you, Reese. Your life has taught me the greatest lessons of love, strength, and endurance. In the hardest moments in our lives, you inspire me to do and be better. As a pediatric nurse practitioner, I questioned my calling prior to having you. Reese, you are my "why" and my muse. Your story motivates me to try harder when I begin to question my abilities. Reese, you are awesome, smart, kind, and strong. Mommy and Daddy love you unconditionally, and eternally.

Love, Alita-Geri (Mommy)

Reese was sick, her parents would have to bring her to the hospital to meet some new friends in the emergency room. When Reese arrived, she noticed the yellow gown with pink bunnies on it, lying on the bed. When she looked around the room, she saw rainbows painted on the walls, and pictures of teddy bears on the ceiling.

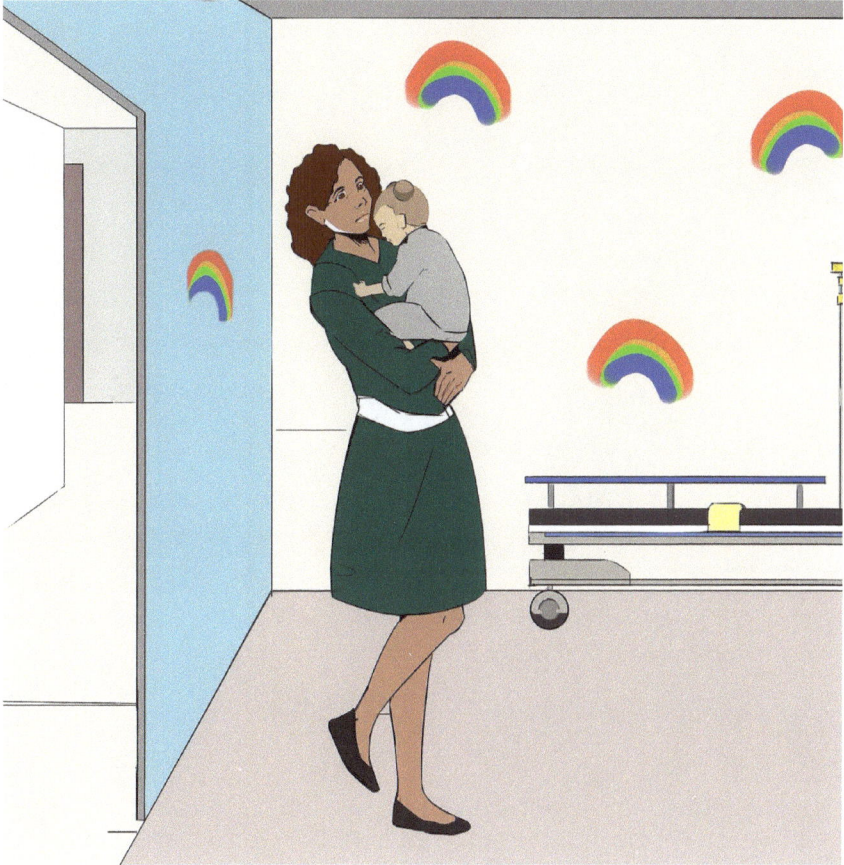

When she put on her gown, the nurse and doctor knew she was ready to meet them. The door to Reese's hospital room opened after a knock and two women appeared.

"Hello Reese! I am Nurse Great!"
"Hello Reese! I am Dr. STEAM!"

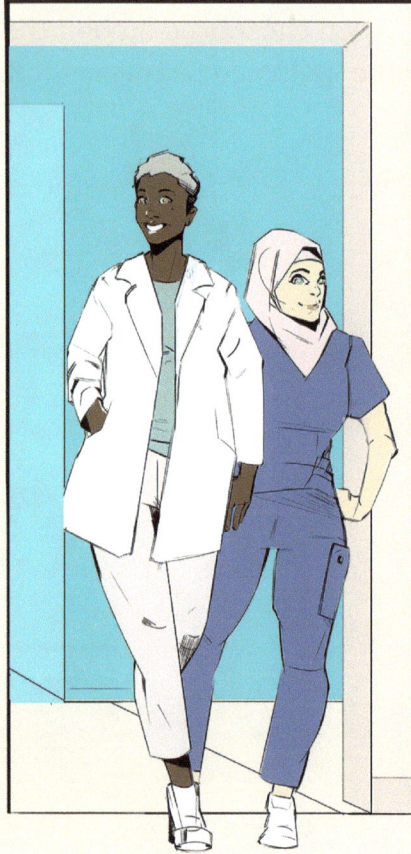

They listened to Reese's chest, back, and tummy with a plastic tube that had a circle at the end called a stethoscope. They tickled her a bit as they listened. Nurse Great and Dr. Steam took turns saying "Ahhh" so Reese could see their teeth. Next, they asked Reese to say "Ahhh." She opened her mouth very wide and made the "Ahhh" sound.

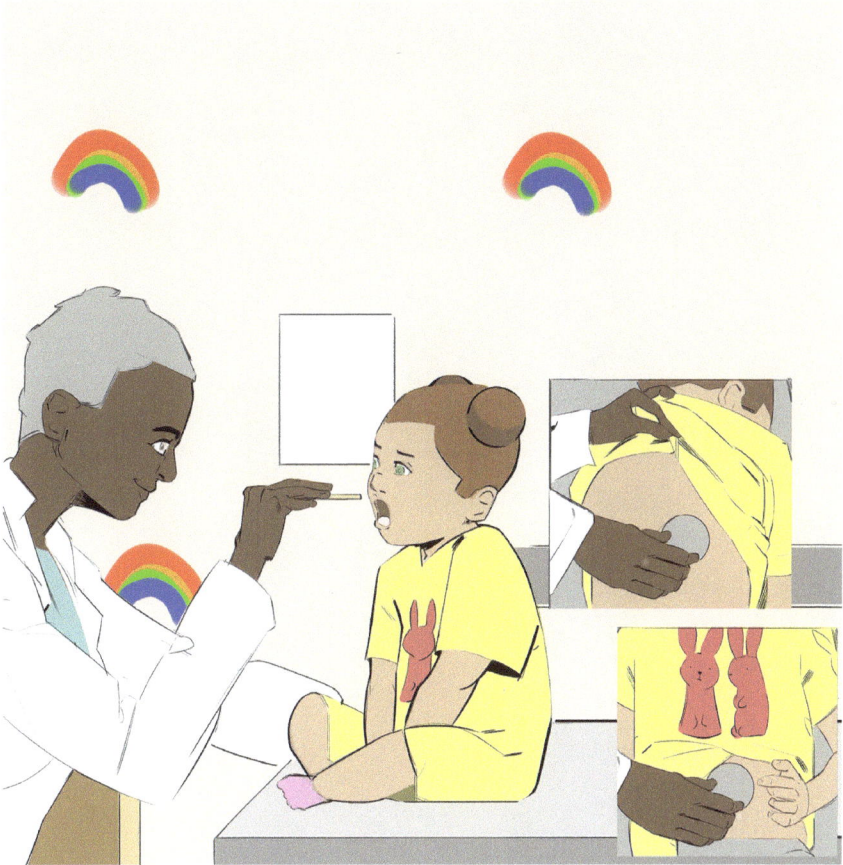

After that, Nurse Great came back to give Reese medicine. Reese sipped the medicine; it did not taste good. Reese sipped some juice afterward to help get rid of the taste. Next, Reese needed to have a picture taken called an X-ray.

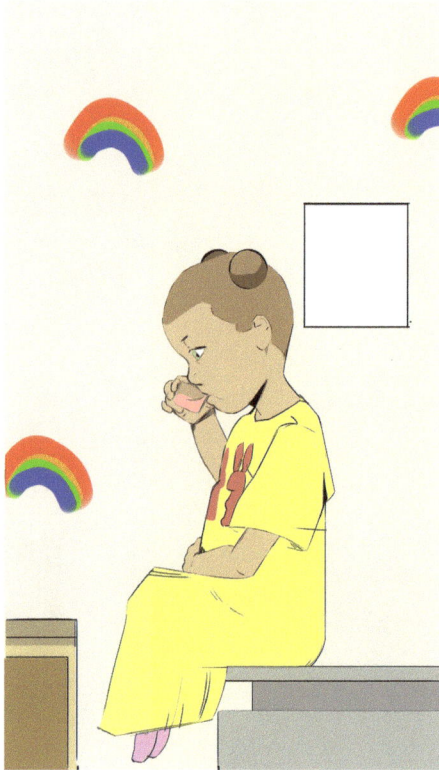

Reese was scared. Reese's mom and dad said, "It is okay to be scared because everyone is afraid at times. We will help you be brave and stay in the room with you during the x-ray picture." It was time for the X-ray. Reese's daddy carried her to the room where there was a huge machine.

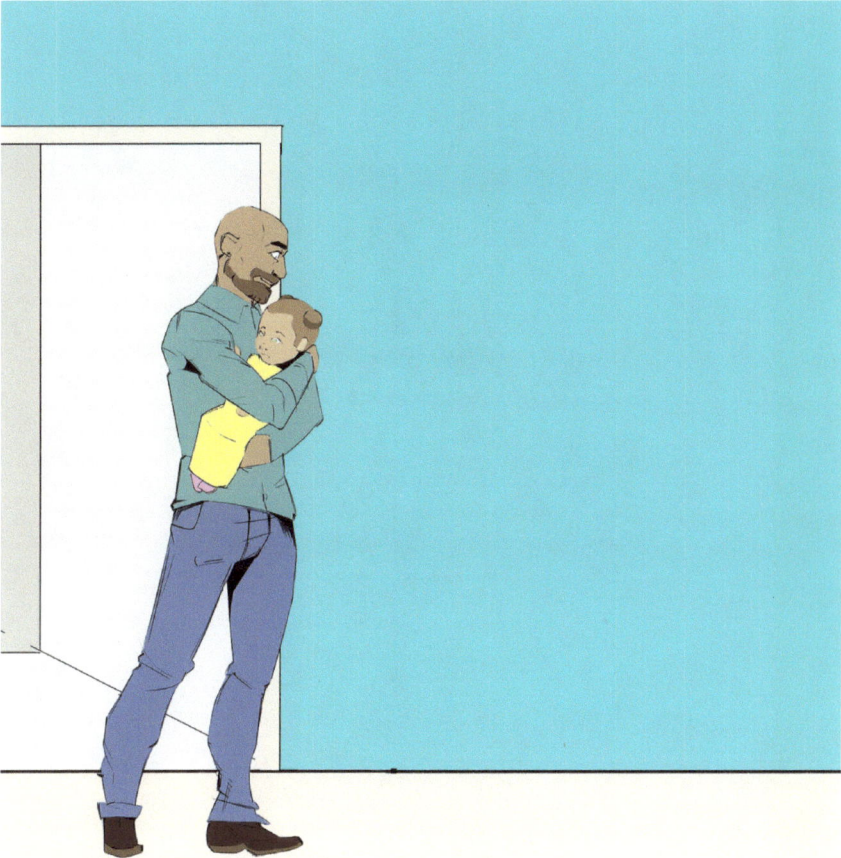

When they entered the room the machine scared Reese. Maria, the lady who would be working the machine, came inside to speak to Reese. "Hi Reese, I am your new friend, Maria and I have a surprise for you".

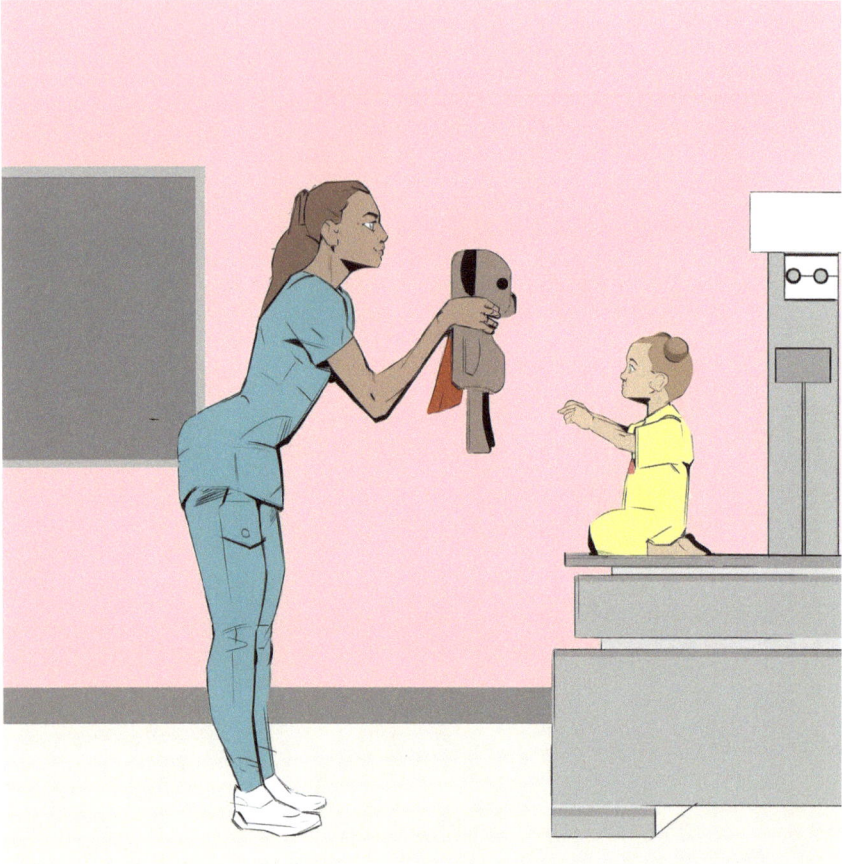

She handed Reese a stuffed puppy that wore a long, red cape. Reese was still scared but her daddy said, "Your new puppy will help you to be brave because you are a superhero too". Reese looked at her new stuffed puppy and decided to be brave too.

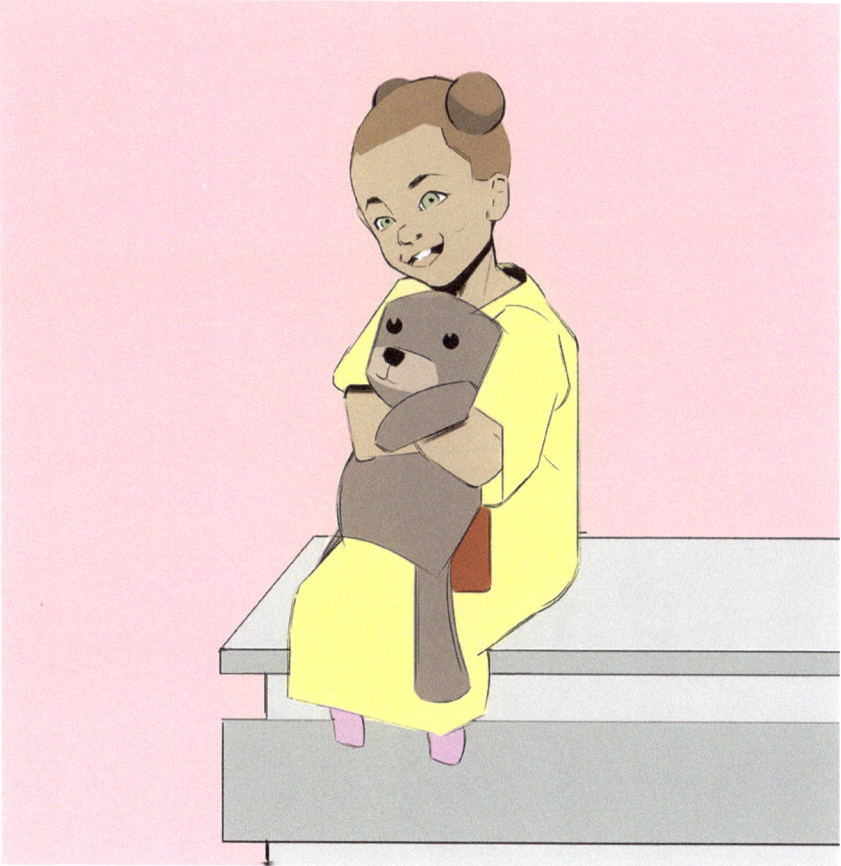

Reese smiled when Maria finished taking her X-ray picture. Reese was beginning to feel better. When she returned to her room, she got a red, strawberry-flavored popsicle. Reese told her parents the name of the dog, "His name is Rufus." Reese and Rufus were now ready to go home. Reese's mom and dad helped her to get dressed. Reese thanked the nurse, and the doctor. "Thank you Nurse Great and Dr. Steam". Reese hugged Rufus and they left the hospital to go home.

THE END

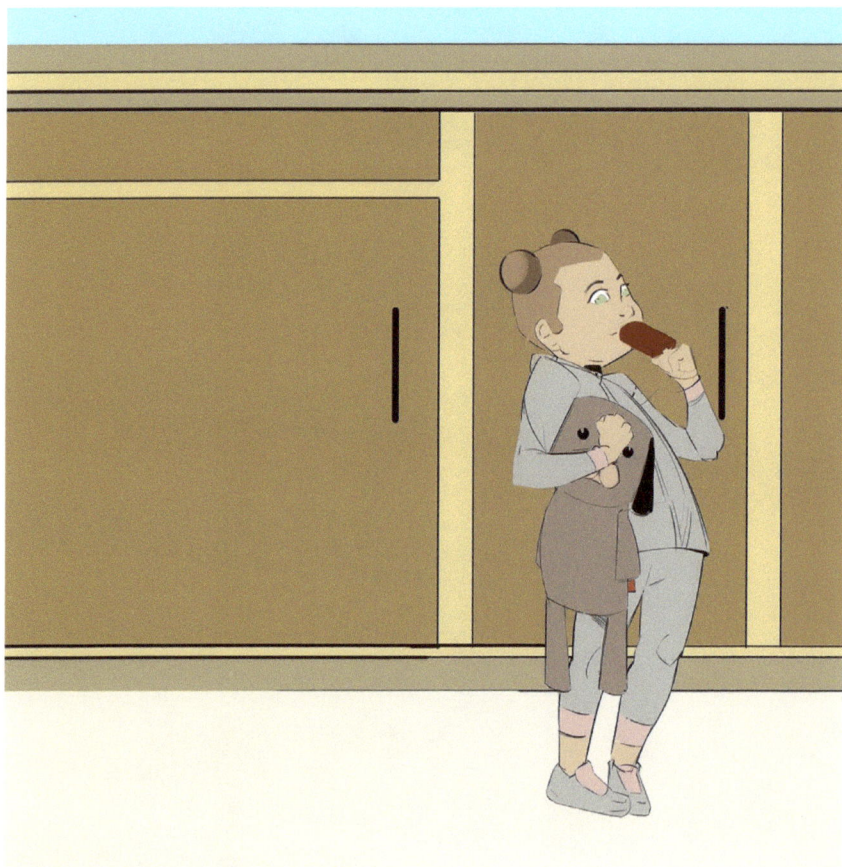

Photograph of Reese leaving a hospital with Rufus and her
Daddy in January of 2018

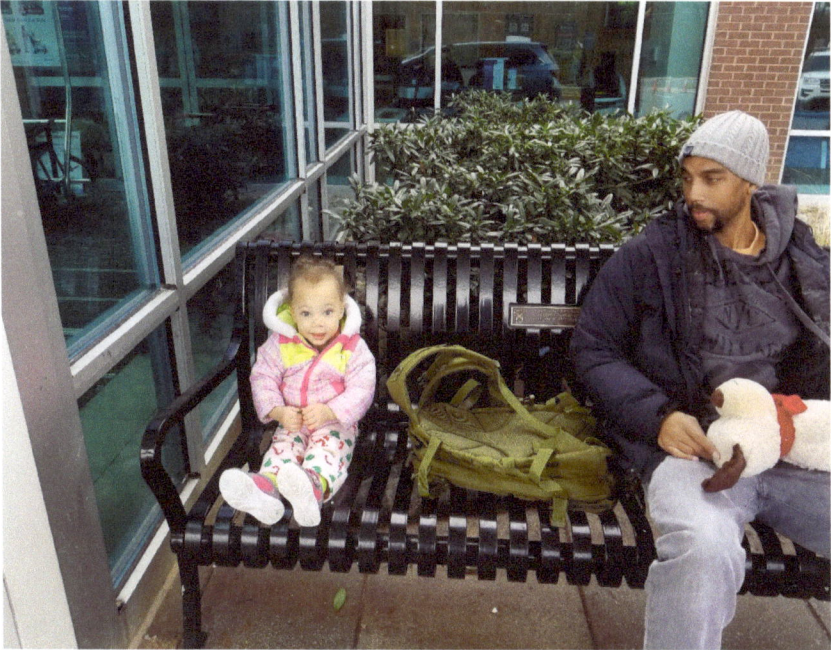

MORE STORIES TO COME
REESE USES THE POTTY
REESE VISITS THE DENTIST
COUNTING PARTS OF THE BODY
Like us on Facebook @ReeseandRufus

COLORING PAGES

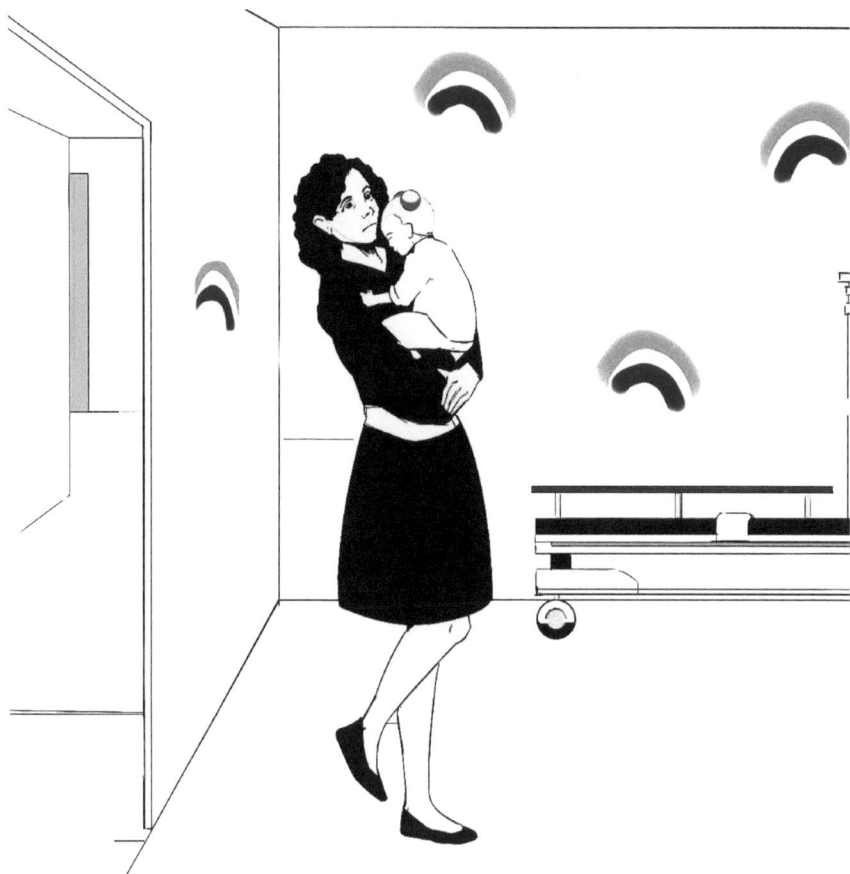

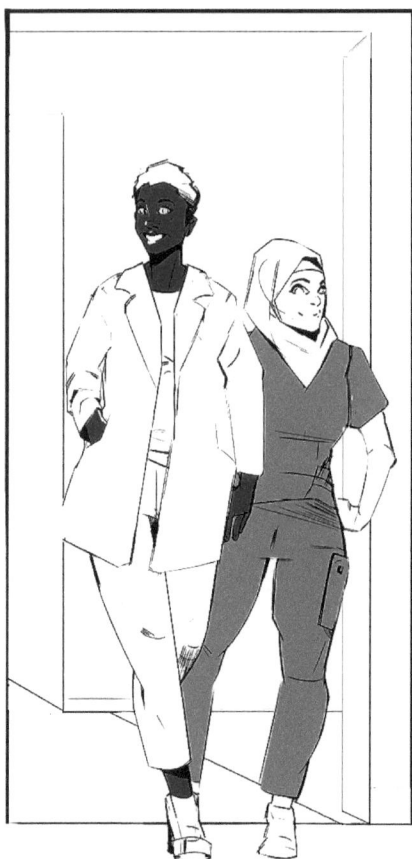

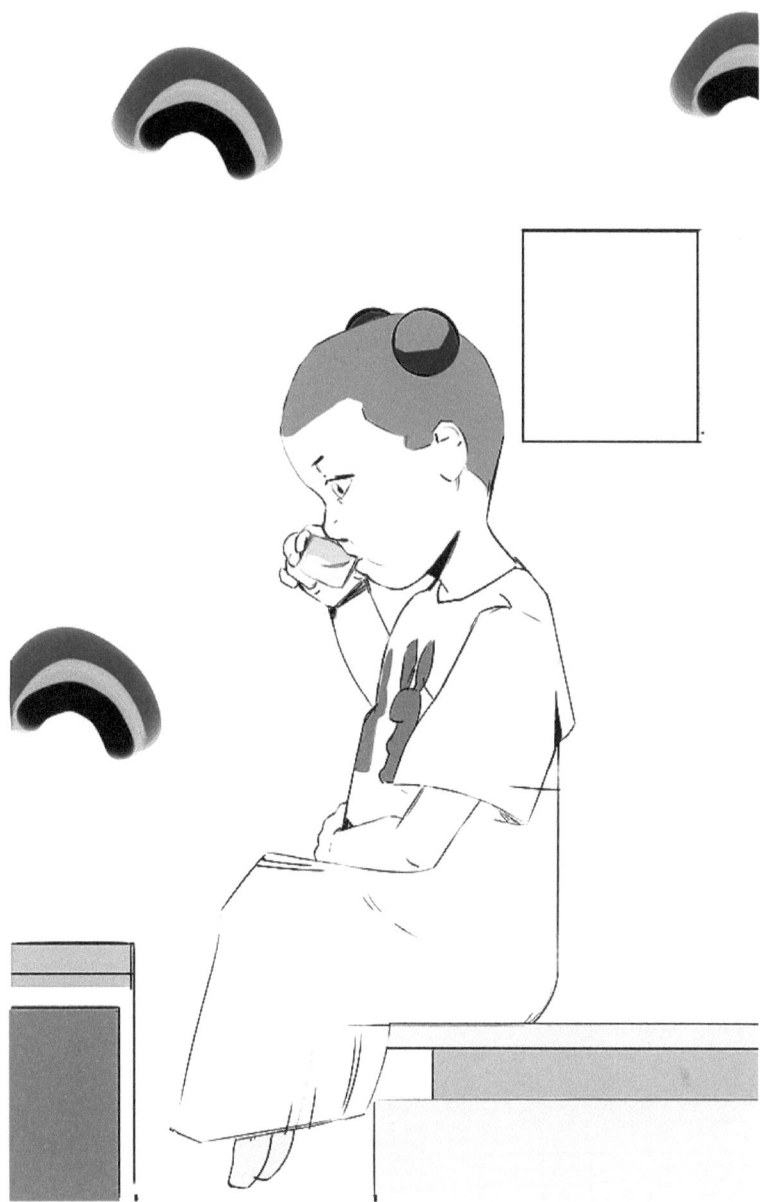

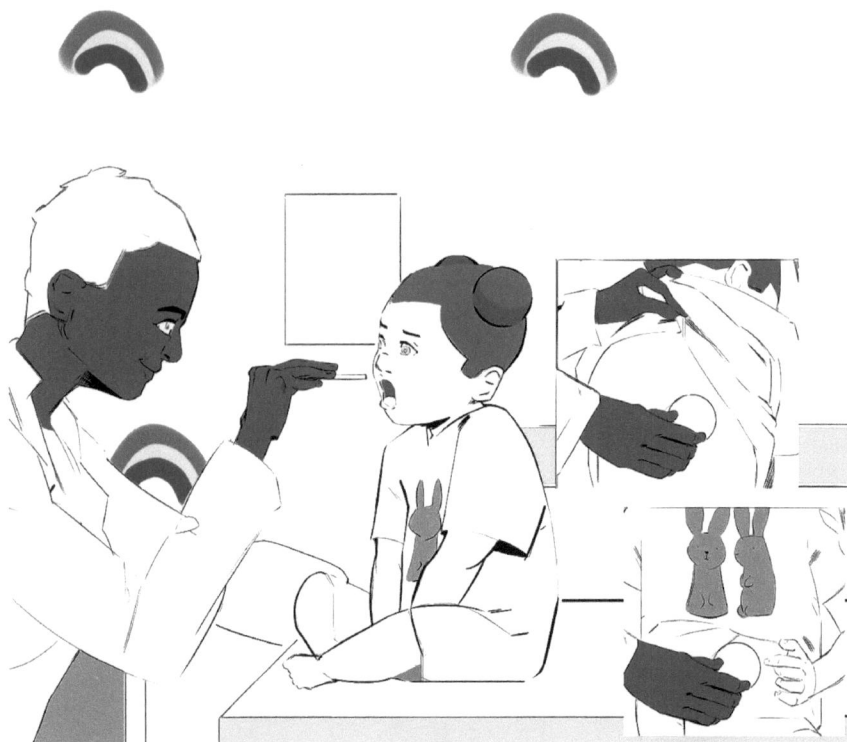

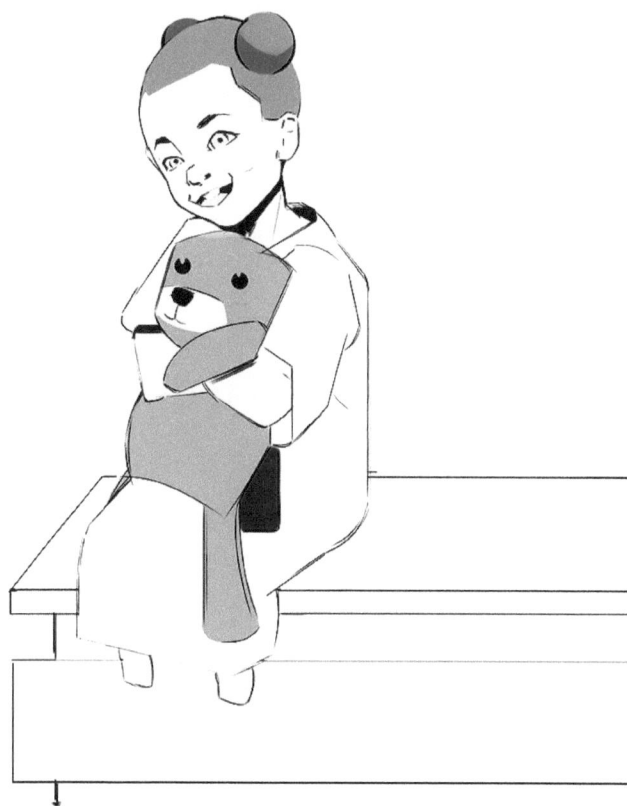

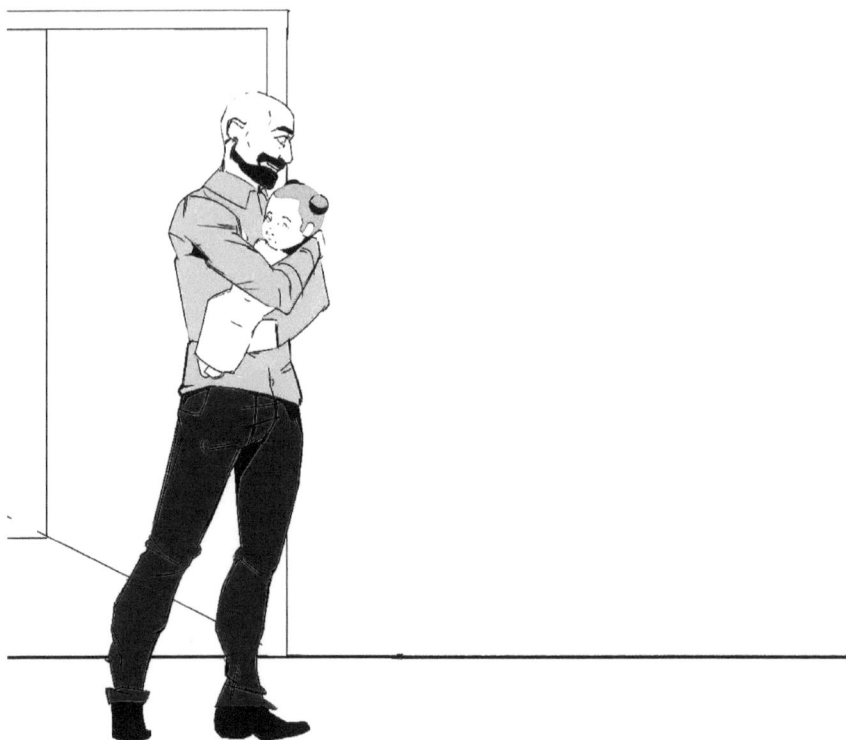

www.ingramcontent.com/pod-product-compliance
Lightning Source LLC
Chambersburg PA
CBHW040932030426
42336CB00001B/11